This Essential Oils Journal Belongs To:

_____

Essential Oil Inventory

NAME	USED FOR	DATE OPENED	FAVORITE?

Essential Oil Wish List

NAME	USED FOR	PRICE	KID SAFE?

My Favorite Oils

ENERGY

CALMING

SLEEP

FOCUS/CLARITY

WELLNESS

ROMANCE

ANXIETY

JOYFUL

Testing Out Blends

NAME:

INGREDIENTS:

PURPOSE:

DIFFUSER

INHALER

TOPICAL

OTHER

MY RATING:

NOTES:

My Oil Ratings

PURPOSE OF OIL

NAME:

MY RATING:

PURPOSE OF OIL

NAME:

MY RATING:

PURPOSE OF OIL

NAME:

MY RATING:

PURPOSE OF OIL

NAME:

MY RATING:

PURPOSE OF OIL

NAME:

MY RATING:

NOTES:

My Favorite Blends

NAME:

USED FOR:

INGREDIENTS:

NOTES:

NAME:

USED FOR:

INGREDIENTS:

NOTES:

My Favorite Blends

NAME: USED FOR:

INGREDIENTS:

NOTES:

NAME: USED FOR:

INGREDIENTS:

NOTES:

Lavender Blends

DIFFUSER BLENDS

NAME: SEA BREEZE

2 DROPS LAVENDER

3 DROPS LIME

1 DROP SPEARMINT

NAME: COOL DOWN

4 DROPS SPEARMINT

2 DROPS LAVENDER

2 DROPS PEPPERMINT

NAME: PEACEFULNESS

3 DROPS LAVENDER

3 DROPS VETIVER

2 DROPS YLANG YLANG

NAME: CREATIVE SPARK

3 DROPS LAVENDER

3 DROPS SWEET ORANGE

1 DROP PEPPERMINT

NAME: OCEAN BREEZE:

4 DROPS LAVENDER

3 DROPS ROSEMARY

2 DROPS LEMONGRASS

NAME: LAVENDAR MINT

4 DROPS LAVENDER

3 DROPS PEPPERMINT

1 DROP VETIVER

NAME: CLEAN AIR

3 DROPS LAVENDER

3 DROPS TANGERINE

3 DROPS EUCALYPTUS

NAME: MINDFULNESS

2 DROPS LAVENDER

3 DROPS BERGAMOT

2 DROPS ROSEMARY

NOTES:

Wellness Blends

DIFFUSER BLENDS

NAME: ENERGIZING

4 DROPS PEPPERMINT

4 DROPS CINNAMON

2 DROPS ROSEMARY

NAME: EXTREME FOCUS

4 DROPS BALANCE

2 DROPS FRANKINCENSE

2 DROPS VETIVER

NAME: INNER CALM

3 DROPS ELEVATION

3 DROPS BERGAMOT

3 DROPS FRANKINCENSE

NAME: TRANQUILITY

3 DROPS LAVENDER

2 DROPS LIME

3 DROPS MANDARIN

NAME: LOVER OF LIFE

3 DROPS ROSEMARY

3 DROPS PEPPERMINT

3 DROPS FRANKINCENSE

NAME: STRESS BE GONE

3 DROPS LAVENDER

2 DROPS CHAMOMILE

2 DROPS YLANG YLANG

NAME: RELAXATION

3 DROPS BERGAMOT

3 DROPS PATCHOULI

3 DROPS YLANG YLANG

NAME: ACTIVE LIFE

2 DROPS GRAPEFRUIT

3 DROPS PEPPERMINT

3 DROPS ROSEMARY

NOTES:

Happiness Blends

DIFFUSER BLENDS

NAME: CHEERFUL
- 3 DROPS WILD ORANGE
- 3 DROPS FRANKINCENSE
- 1 DROP CINNAMON

NAME: SWEETNESS
- 3 DROPS BERGAMOT
- 2 DROPS GERANIUM
- 3 DROPS LAVENDER

NAME: INNER PEACE
- 2 DROPS PEPPERMINT
- 2 DROPS LAVENDER
- 2 DROPS WILD ORANGE

NAME: ZONED OUT
- 2 DROPS ROSEMARY
- 2 DROPS CINNAMON
- 1 DROP CLOVE

NAME: WITH PURPOSE
- 3 DROPS LEMON
- 2 DROPS OREGANO
- 2 DROPS ON GUARD

NAME: LAUGHTER
- 3 DROPS LEMON
- 3 DROPS TANGERINE
- 2 DROPS MELALEUCA

NAME: BOOSTER
- 2 DROPS LAVENDER
- 3 DROPS SWEET ORANGE
- 3 DROPS PEPPERMINT

NAME: MINDFULNESS
- 3 DROPS LAVENDER
- 3 DROPS BERGAMOT
- 1 DROP CLOVE

NOTES:

Well Rested Blends

DIFFUSER BLENDS

NAME: WELL RESTED

3 DROPS JUNIPER BERRY

3 DROPS CHAMOMILE

3 DROPS LAVENDER

NAME: WELL RESTED 2

4 DROPS CEDARWOOD

3 DROPS LAVENDER

1 DROP VETIVER

NAME: WELL RESTED 3

2 DROPS FRANKINCENSE

3 DROPS VETIVER

2 DROPS LAVENDER

NAME: WELL RESTED 4

3 DROPS BALANCE

2 DROPS LAVENDER

2 DROPS CHAMOMILE

NAME: WELL RESTED 5

3 DROPS LAVENDER

2 DROPS MARJORAM

2 DROPS ORANGE

NAME: WELL RESTED 6

3 DROPS LEMON

3 DROPS LAVENDER

2 DROPS PEPPERMINT

NAME: WELL RESTED 7

5 DROPS PEPPERMINT

4 DROPS EUCALYPTUS

2 DROPS MYRRH

NAME: WELL RESTED 8

3 DROPS LAVENDER

3 DROPS CHAMOMILE

1 DROP CLOVE

NOTES:

Autumn Blends

DIFFUSER BLENDS

NAME: PUMPKIN SPICE

5 DROPS CINNAMON

2 DROPS NUTMEG

3 DROPS CLOVE

NAME: SNICKERDOODLE

5 DROPS STRESS AWAY

3 DROPS CINNAMON

2 DROPS NUTMEG

NAME: FLANNEL SHEETS

5 DROPS BLACK SPRUCE

4 DROPS STRESS AWAY

4 DROPS ORANGE

NAME: SWEATER WEATHER

5 DROPS ORANGE

4 DROPS THIEVES

1 DROP GINGER

NAME: CIDER

4 DROPS ORANGE

3 DROPS CINNAMON

3 DROPS GINGER

NAME: CHANGING LEAVES

5 DROPS CLOVE

5 DROPS CEDARWOOD

5 DROPS ORANGE

NAME: GIVING THANKS

5 DROPS CINNAMON

3 DROPS ORANGE

2 DROPS NUTMEG

NAME: AUTUMN BREEZE

5 DROPS CHRISTMAS SPIRIT

2 DROPS CLOVE

1 DROP LEMON

NOTES:

Summer Blends

DIFFUSER BLENDS

NAME: SWEET SUNSHINE

3 DROPS LEMONGRASS

2 DROPS ORANGE

1 DROP PEPPERMINT

NAME: SUNNY DAYS

3 DROPS TANGERINE

3 DROPS LEMON

1 DROP PEPPERMINT

NAME: HAMMOCK TIME

2 DROPS LAVENDER

2 DROPS CEDARWOOD

2 DROPS WILD ORANGE

NAME: CITRUS TWIST

2 DROPS TANGERINE

2 DROPS GRAPEFRUIT

2 DROPS LEMON

NAME: SUMMER LOVING

2 DROPS JUNIPER BERRY

2 DROPS GRAPEFRUIT

2 DROPS WILD ORANGE

NAME: OCEAN BREEZE

3 DROPS BERGAMOT

3 DROPS LAVENDER

3 DROPS ROSEMARY

NAME: BEACH MEMORIES

2 DROPS SPEARMINT

3 DROPS TANGERINE

2 DROPS BERGAMOT

NAME: SUN KISSED

2 DROPS TEA TREE

2 DROPS LEMON

2 DROPS LIME

NOTES:

Winter Blends

DIFFUSER BLENDS

NAME: WINTER CITRUS

2 DROPS PEPPERMINT

2 DROPS LEMONGRASS

2 DROPS TANGERINE

NAME: CLASSIC WINTER

2 DROPS CEDARWOOD

2 DROPS LAVENDER

2 DROPS ROSEMARY

NAME: SNOWFLAKE

2 DROPS LAVENDER

2 DROPS LEMON

2 DROPS DIGIZE

NAME: HOLIDAY BAKING

2 DROPS CASSIA

2 DROPS VETIVER

2 DROPS LAVENDAR

NAME: SNOW DAYS

2 DROPS STRESS AWAY

2 DROPS THIEVES

2 DROPS CITRUS

NAME: COZY HOME

2 DROPS BERGAMOT

2 DROPS ORANGE

2 DROPS THIEVES

NAME: MOTHER NATURE

3 DROPS PEPPERMINT

3 DROPS LAVENDER

3 DROPS LEMON

NAME: WINTER MEMORIES

2 DROPS BERGAMOT

2 DROPS WILD ORANGE

2 DROPS EUCALYPTUS

NOTES:

Spring Blends

DIFFUSER BLENDS

NAME: WELCOME SPRING

2 DROPS GERANIUM

2 DROPS LEMON

2 DROPS GRAPEFRUIT

NAME: FRESH & CLEAN

4 DROPS GRAPEFRUIT

3 DROPS PEPPERMINT

3 DROPS CLARY SAGE

NAME: SPRING PETALS

2 DROPS YLANG YLANG

2 DROPS PEPPERMINT

2 DROPS JADE LEMON

NAME: SPRING CLEANING

2 DROPS LAVENDAR

3 DROPS LEMON

3 DROPS ROSEMARY

NAME: SPRING GARDEN

2 DROPS BASIL

2 DROPS PEPPERMINT

2 DROPS LIME

NAME: FRESH FLOWERS

5 DROPS CLARY SAGE

3 DROPS LAVENDAR

2 DROPS GERANIUM

NAME: MOTHER NATURE

3 DROPS PEPPERMINT

3 DROPS LAVENDAR

3 DROPS LEMON

NAME: GOOD MORNING

4 DROPS JOY

3 DROPS LEMON

1 DROP TANGERINE

NOTES:

Holiday Blends

DIFFUSER BLENDS

NAME: DECK THE HALLS

4 DROPS PINE

2 DROPS BLUE SPRUCE

2 DROPS CEDARWOOD

NAME: CANDY CANE

4 DROPS PEPPERMINT

3 DROPS BERGAMOT

1 DROP WILD ORANGE

NAME: SUGAR PLUM FAIRY

3 DROPS CITRUS BLISS

2 DROPS DOUGLAS FIR

2 DROPS MOTIVATE

NAME: OH, HOLY NIGHT

5 DROPS THIEVES

2 DROPS FRANKINCENSE

2 DROPS CITRUS FRESH

NAME: SNOW ANGELS

4 DROPS STRESS AWAY

3 FRESH CITRUS

1 DROP FRANKINCENSE

NAME: SPICED CIDER

3 DROPS WILD ORANGE

2 DROPS CINNAMON BARK

1 DROP CLOVE

NAME: MERRY & BRIGHT

3 DROPS LEMON

2 DROPS DOUGLAS FIR

2 DROPS CINNAMON

NAME: GINGERBREAD MAN

4 DROPS GINGER

2 DROPS CLOVES

2 DROPS CINNAMON

NOTES:

Clean House Blends

DIFFUSER BLENDS

NAME: SPARKLY CLEAN

3 DROPS LEMON

3 DROPS PEPPERMINT

3 DROPS EUCALYPTUS

NAME: NICE & TIDY

3 DROPS EUCALYPTUS

3 DROPS WILD ORANGE

3 DROPS LIME

NAME: FRESH SCENT

3 DROPS LEMON

3 DROPS EASY AIR

3 DROPS LIME

NAME: TIDY HOME

1 DROP ROSE

1 DROP CARDAMOM

2 DROPS WILD ORANGE

NAME: DECLUTTERING

4 DROPS LEMON

3 DROPS LEMONGRASS

2 DROPS PEPPERMINT

NAME: SPRING CLEANING

4 DROPS LEMON

3 DROPS LAVENDER

2 DROPS ROSEMARY

NAME: GLOSSY CLEAN

4 DROPS FRANKINCENSE

4 DROPS CYPRESS

2 DROPS YLANG YLANG

NAME: HOUSEKEEPER

2 DROPS CINNAMON

2 DROPS CARDAMOM

2 DROPS LEMOM

NOTES:

Personality Blends

DIFFUSER BLENDS

NAME: CONFIDENT

2 DROPS SPEARMINT

2 DROPS TANGERINE

2 DROPS BERGAMOT

NAME: CAREFREE

5 DROPS BERGAMOT

2 DROPS PATCHOULI

2 DROPS LIME

NAME: HAPPY

2 DROPS WILD ORANGE

2 DROPS GRAPEFRUIT

2 DROPS CLOVE

NAME: INSPIRED

1 DROP ROSE

1 DROP PURIFY

2 DROPS JUNIPER BERRY

NAME: FOCUSED

3 DROPS DOUGLAS FIR

2 DROPS LEMON

1 DROP PEPPERMINT

NAME: ENERGETIC

2 DROPS PEPPERMINT

3 DROPS GRAPEFRUIT

3 DROPS BERGAMOT

NAME: MOTIVATED

2 DROPS ELEVATION

2 DROPS CYPRESS

2 DROPS LIME

NAME: PEACEFUL

2 DROPS FRANKINCENSE

2 DROPS WHITE FIR

2 DROPS LAVENDER

NOTES:

Day to Day Blends

DIFFUSER BLENDS

NAME: SLEEP TIME

4 DROPS LAVENDER

4 DROPS CEDARWOOD

3 DROPS CHAMOMILE

NAME: ANTI-STRESS

4 DROPS BERGAMOT

4 DROPS FRANKINCENSE

1 DROP PEPPERMINT

NAME: ALLERGY BE GONE

3 DROPS LAVENDER

3 DROPS LEMON

3 DROPS PEPPERMINT

NAME: CONCENTRATION

4 DROPS LAVENDER

4 DROPS MELALEUCA

4 DROPS FRANKINCENSE

NAME: COMBAT NAUSEA

3 DROPS GINGER

5 DROPS PEPPERMINT

1 DROP BALANCE

NAME: HEADACHES

2 DROPS FRANKINCENSE

2 DROPS LAVENDER

4 DROPS PEPPERMINT

NAME: BREATHE EASY

4 DROPS PEPPERMINT

2 DROPS EUCALYPTUS

2 DROPS LEMON

NAME: IMMUNE BOOST

2 DROPS FRANKINCENSE

5 DROPS LEMON

2 DROPS PEPPERMINT

NOTES:

Essential Oil Recipes

NAME:

NAME:

NAME:

NAME:

NAME:

NAME:

NAME:

NAME:

Essential Oil Recipes

NAME:

NAME:

NAME:

NAME:

NAME:

NAME:

NAME:

NAME:

Essential Oil Wish List

NAME	USED FOR	PRICE	KID SAFE?

My Favorite Oils

ENERGY

CALMING

SLEEP

FOCUS/CLARITY

WELLNESS

ROMANCE

ANXIETY

JOYFUL

Essential Oil Inventory

NAME	USED FOR	DATE OPENED	FAVORITE?

My Favorite Blends

NAME: USED FOR:

INGREDIENTS:

NOTES:

NAME: USED FOR:

INGREDIENTS:

NOTES:

Essential Oil Inventory

NAME	USED FOR	DATE OPENED	FAVORITE?

Essential Oil Wish List

NAME	USED FOR	PRICE	KID SAFE?

My Favorite Oils

ENERGY

CALMING

SLEEP

FOCUS/CLARITY

WELLNESS

ROMANCE

ANXIETY

JOYFUL

Testing Out Blends

NAME:

INGREDIENTS:

PURPOSE:

DIFFUSER

INHALER

TOPICAL

OTHER

MY RATING:

NOTES:

Testing Out Blends

NAME:

PURPOSE:

INGREDIENTS:

DIFFUSER

INHALER

TOPICAL

OTHER

MY RATING:

NOTES:

Testing Out Blends

NAME:

INGREDIENTS:

PURPOSE:

DIFFUSER

INHALER

TOPICAL

OTHER

MY RATING:

NOTES:

Testing Out Blends

NAME:

PURPOSE:

INGREDIENTS:

DIFFUSER

INHALER

TOPICAL

OTHER

MY RATING:

NOTES:

My Oil Ratings

PURPOSE OF OIL

NAME:

MY RATING:

PURPOSE OF OIL

NAME:

MY RATING:

PURPOSE OF OIL

NAME:

MY RATING:

PURPOSE OF OIL

NAME:

MY RATING:

PURPOSE OF OIL

NAME:

MY RATING:

NOTES:

My Oil Ratings

PURPOSE OF OIL

NAME:

MY RATING:

PURPOSE OF OIL

NAME:

MY RATING:

PURPOSE OF OIL

NAME:

MY RATING:

PURPOSE OF OIL

NAME:

MY RATING:

PURPOSE OF OIL

NAME:

MY RATING:

NOTES:

My Oil Ratings

PURPOSE OF OIL

NAME:

MY RATING:

PURPOSE OF OIL

NAME:

MY RATING:

PURPOSE OF OIL

NAME:

MY RATING:

PURPOSE OF OIL

NAME:

MY RATING:

PURPOSE OF OIL

NAME:

MY RATING:

NOTES:

My Favorite Blends

NAME:

INGREDIENTS:

USED FOR:

NOTES:

NAME:

INGREDIENTS:

USED FOR:

NOTES:

My Favorite Blends

NAME:

USED FOR:

INGREDIENTS:

NOTES:

NAME:

USED FOR:

INGREDIENTS:

NOTES:

My Favorite Blends

NAME:

USED FOR:

INGREDIENTS:

NOTES:

NAME:

USED FOR:

INGREDIENTS:

NOTES:

My Favorite Blends

NAME: **USED FOR:**

INGREDIENTS:

NOTES:

NAME: **USED FOR:**

INGREDIENTS:

NOTES:

Essential Oil Inventory

NAME	USED FOR	DATE OPENED	FAVORITE?

Essential Oil Wish List

NAME	USED FOR	PRICE	KID SAFE?

My Favorite Oils

ENERGY

CALMING

SLEEP

FOCUS/CLARITY

WELLNESS

ROMANCE

ANXIETY

JOYFUL

Testing Out Blends

NAME:

PURPOSE:

INGREDIENTS:

DIFFUSER

INHALER

TOPICAL

OTHER

MY RATING:

NOTES:

My Oil Ratings

PURPOSE OF OIL

NAME:

MY RATING:

PURPOSE OF OIL

NAME:

MY RATING:

PURPOSE OF OIL

NAME:

MY RATING:

PURPOSE OF OIL

NAME:

MY RATING:

PURPOSE OF OIL

NAME:

MY RATING:

NOTES:

My Favorite Blends

NAME: USED FOR:

INGREDIENTS:

NOTES:

NAME: USED FOR:

INGREDIENTS:

NOTES:

My Favorite Blends

NAME: **USED FOR:**

INGREDIENTS:

NOTES:

NAME: **USED FOR:**

INGREDIENTS:

NOTES:

Essential Oil Inventory

NAME	USED FOR	DATE OPENED	FAVORITE?

Essential Oil Wish List

NAME	USED FOR	PRICE	KID SAFE?

My Favorite Oils

ENERGY

CALMING

SLEEP

FOCUS/CLARITY

WELLNESS

ROMANCE

ANXIETY

JOYFUL

Testing Out Blends

NAME:

INGREDIENTS:

PURPOSE:

DIFFUSER

INHALER

TOPICAL

OTHER

MY RATING:

NOTES:

My Oil Ratings

PURPOSE OF OIL

NAME:

MY RATING:

PURPOSE OF OIL

NAME:

MY RATING:

PURPOSE OF OIL

NAME:

MY RATING:

PURPOSE OF OIL

NAME:

MY RATING:

PURPOSE OF OIL

NAME:

MY RATING:

NOTES:

My Favorite Blends

NAME:

USED FOR:

INGREDIENTS:

NOTES:

NAME:

USED FOR:

INGREDIENTS:

NOTES:

My Favorite Blends

NAME: USED FOR:

INGREDIENTS:

NOTES:

NAME: USED FOR:

INGREDIENTS:

NOTES:

Essential Oil Inventory

NAME	USED FOR	DATE OPENED	FAVORITE?

Essential Oil Wish List

NAME	USED FOR	PRICE	KID SAFE?

My Favorite Oils

ENERGY

CALMING

SLEEP

FOCUS/CLARITY

WELLNESS

ROMANCE

ANXIETY

JOYFUL

Testing Out Blends

NAME:

PURPOSE:

INGREDIENTS:

DIFFUSER

INHALER

TOPICAL

OTHER

MY RATING:

NOTES:

My Oil Ratings

PURPOSE OF OIL

NAME:

MY RATING:

PURPOSE OF OIL

NAME:

MY RATING:

PURPOSE OF OIL

NAME:

MY RATING:

PURPOSE OF OIL

NAME:

MY RATING:

PURPOSE OF OIL

NAME:

MY RATING:

NOTES:

My Favorite Blends

NAME: USED FOR:

INGREDIENTS:

NOTES:

NAME: USED FOR:

INGREDIENTS:

NOTES:

My Favorite Blends

NAME:

INGREDIENTS:

USED FOR:

NOTES:

NAME:

INGREDIENTS:

USED FOR:

NOTES:

Essential Oil Inventory

NAME	USED FOR	DATE OPENED	FAVORITE?

Essential Oil Wish List

NAME	USED FOR	PRICE	KID SAFE?

My Favorite Oils

ENERGY

CALMING

SLEEP

FOCUS/CLARITY

WELLNESS

ROMANCE

ANXIETY

JOYFUL

Testing Out Blends

NAME:

INGREDIENTS:

PURPOSE:

DIFFUSER

INHALER

TOPICAL

OTHER

MY RATING:

NOTES:

My Oil Ratings

PURPOSE OF OIL

NAME:

MY RATING:

PURPOSE OF OIL

NAME:

MY RATING:

PURPOSE OF OIL

NAME:

MY RATING:

PURPOSE OF OIL

NAME:

MY RATING:

PURPOSE OF OIL

NAME:

MY RATING:

NOTES:

My Favorite Blends

NAME:

USED FOR:

INGREDIENTS:

NOTES:

NAME:

USED FOR:

INGREDIENTS:

NOTES:

My Favorite Blends

NAME:

USED FOR:

INGREDIENTS:

NOTES:

NAME:

USED FOR:

INGREDIENTS:

NOTES:

Essential Oil Inventory

NAME	USED FOR	DATE OPENED	FAVORITE?

Essential Oil Wish List

NAME	USED FOR	PRICE	KID SAFE?

My Favorite Oils

ENERGY

CALMING

SLEEP

FOCUS/CLARITY

WELLNESS

ROMANCE

ANXIETY

JOYFUL

Testing Out Blends

NAME:

PURPOSE:

INGREDIENTS:

- DIFFUSER
- INHALER
- TOPICAL
- OTHER

MY RATING:

NOTES:

My Oil Ratings

PURPOSE OF OIL

NAME:

MY RATING:

PURPOSE OF OIL

NAME:

MY RATING:

PURPOSE OF OIL

NAME:

MY RATING:

PURPOSE OF OIL

NAME:

MY RATING:

PURPOSE OF OIL

NAME:

MY RATING:

NOTES:

My Favorite Blends

NAME:

USED FOR:

INGREDIENTS:

NOTES:

NAME:

USED FOR:

INGREDIENTS:

NOTES:

My Favorite Blends

NAME:

INGREDIENTS:

USED FOR:

NOTES:

NAME:

INGREDIENTS:

USED FOR:

NOTES:

Essential Oil Inventory

NAME	USED FOR	DATE OPENED	FAVORITE?

Essential Oil Wish List

NAME	USED FOR	PRICE	KID SAFE?

My Favorite Oils

ENERGY

CALMING

SLEEP

FOCUS/CLARITY

WELLNESS

ROMANCE

ANXIETY

JOYFUL

Testing Out Blends

NAME:

INGREDIENTS:

PURPOSE:

DIFFUSER

INHALER

TOPICAL

OTHER

MY RATING:

NOTES:

My Oil Ratings

PURPOSE OF OIL

NAME:

MY RATING:

PURPOSE OF OIL

NAME:

MY RATING:

PURPOSE OF OIL

NAME:

MY RATING:

PURPOSE OF OIL

NAME:

MY RATING:

PURPOSE OF OIL

NAME:

MY RATING:

NOTES:

My Favorite Blends

NAME:

USED FOR:

INGREDIENTS:

NOTES:

NAME:

USED FOR:

INGREDIENTS:

NOTES:

My Favorite Blends

NAME:

USED FOR:

INGREDIENTS:

NOTES:

NAME:

USED FOR:

INGREDIENTS:

NOTES:

Essential Oil Inventory

NAME	USED FOR	DATE OPENED	FAVORITE?

Essential Oil Wish List

NAME	USED FOR	PRICE	KID SAFE?

My Favorite Oils

ENERGY

CALMING

SLEEP

FOCUS/CLARITY

WELLNESS

ROMANCE

ANXIETY

JOYFUL

Testing Out Blends

NAME:

INGREDIENTS:

PURPOSE:

DIFFUSER

INHALER

TOPICAL

OTHER

MY RATING:

NOTES:

My Oil Ratings

PURPOSE OF OIL

NAME:

MY RATING:

PURPOSE OF OIL

NAME:

MY RATING:

PURPOSE OF OIL

NAME:

MY RATING:

PURPOSE OF OIL

NAME:

MY RATING:

PURPOSE OF OIL

NAME:

MY RATING:

NOTES:

My Favorite Blends

NAME:

USED FOR:

INGREDIENTS:

NOTES:

NAME:

USED FOR:

INGREDIENTS:

NOTES:

My Favorite Blends

NAME:

USED FOR:

INGREDIENTS:

NOTES:

NAME:

USED FOR:

INGREDIENTS:

NOTES:

Essential Oil Inventory

NAME	USED FOR	DATE OPENED	FAVORITE?

Essential Oil Wish List

NAME	USED FOR	PRICE	KID SAFE?

My Favorite Oils

ENERGY

CALMING

SLEEP

FOCUS/CLARITY

WELLNESS

ROMANCE

ANXIETY

JOYFUL

Testing Out Blends

NAME:

PURPOSE:

INGREDIENTS:

DIFFUSER

INHALER

TOPICAL

OTHER

MY RATING:

NOTES:

My Oil Ratings

PURPOSE OF OIL

NAME:

MY RATING:

PURPOSE OF OIL

NAME:

MY RATING:

PURPOSE OF OIL

NAME:

MY RATING:

PURPOSE OF OIL

NAME:

MY RATING:

PURPOSE OF OIL

NAME:

MY RATING:

NOTES:

My Favorite Blends

NAME: **USED FOR:**

INGREDIENTS:

NOTES:

NAME: **USED FOR:**

INGREDIENTS:

NOTES:

My Favorite Blends

NAME: **USED FOR:**

INGREDIENTS:

NOTES:

NAME: **USED FOR:**

INGREDIENTS:

NOTES:

Essential Oil Inventory

NAME	USED FOR	DATE OPENED	FAVORITE?

Essential Oil Wish List

NAME	USED FOR	PRICE	KID SAFE?

My Favorite Oils

ENERGY

CALMING

SLEEP

FOCUS/CLARITY

WELLNESS

ROMANCE

ANXIETY

JOYFUL

Testing Out Blends

NAME:

PURPOSE:

INGREDIENTS:

- DIFFUSER
- INHALER
- TOPICAL
- OTHER

MY RATING:

NOTES:

My Oil Ratings

PURPOSE OF OIL

NAME:

MY RATING:

PURPOSE OF OIL

NAME:

MY RATING:

PURPOSE OF OIL

NAME:

MY RATING:

PURPOSE OF OIL

NAME:

MY RATING:

PURPOSE OF OIL

NAME:

MY RATING:

NOTES:

My Favorite Blends

NAME:

USED FOR:

INGREDIENTS:

NOTES:

NAME:

USED FOR:

INGREDIENTS:

NOTES:

My Favorite Blends

NAME:

INGREDIENTS:

USED FOR:

NOTES:

NAME:

INGREDIENTS:

USED FOR:

NOTES:

Essential Oil Inventory

NAME	USED FOR	DATE OPENED	FAVORITE?

Essential Oil Wish List

NAME	USED FOR	PRICE	KID SAFE?

My Favorite Oils

ENERGY

CALMING

SLEEP

FOCUS/CLARITY

WELLNESS

ROMANCE

ANXIETY

JOYFUL

Testing Out Blends

NAME:

PURPOSE:

INGREDIENTS:

DIFFUSER

INHALER

TOPICAL

OTHER

MY RATING:

NOTES:

My Oil Ratings

PURPOSE OF OIL

NAME:

MY RATING:

PURPOSE OF OIL

NAME:

MY RATING:

PURPOSE OF OIL

NAME:

MY RATING:

PURPOSE OF OIL

NAME:

MY RATING:

PURPOSE OF OIL

NAME:

MY RATING:

NOTES:

My Favorite Blends

NAME:

USED FOR:

INGREDIENTS:

NOTES:

NAME:

USED FOR:

INGREDIENTS:

NOTES:

My Favorite Blends

NAME:

USED FOR:

INGREDIENTS:

NOTES:

NAME:

USED FOR:

INGREDIENTS:

NOTES:

Essential Oil Inventory

NAME	USED FOR	DATE OPENED	FAVORITE?

Essential Oil Wish List

NAME	USED FOR	PRICE	KID SAFE?

My Favorite Oils

ENERGY

_____
_____
_____
_____
_____

SLEEP

_____
_____
_____
_____
_____

WELLNESS

_____
_____
_____
_____
_____

ANXIETY

_____
_____
_____
_____
_____

CALMING

_____
_____
_____
_____
_____

FOCUS/CLARITY

_____
_____
_____
_____
_____

ROMANCE

_____
_____
_____
_____
_____

JOYFUL

_____
_____
_____
_____
_____

Testing Out Blends

NAME:

PURPOSE:

INGREDIENTS:

- DIFFUSER
- INHALER
- TOPICAL
- OTHER

MY RATING:

NOTES:

My Oil Ratings

PURPOSE OF OIL

NAME:

MY RATING:

PURPOSE OF OIL

NAME:

MY RATING:

PURPOSE OF OIL

NAME:

MY RATING:

PURPOSE OF OIL

NAME:

MY RATING:

PURPOSE OF OIL

NAME:

MY RATING:

NOTES:

My Favorite Blends

NAME: **USED FOR:**

INGREDIENTS:

NOTES:

NAME: **USED FOR:**

INGREDIENTS:

NOTES:

My Favorite Blends

NAME:

USED FOR:

INGREDIENTS:

NOTES:

NAME:

USED FOR:

INGREDIENTS:

NOTES:

Essential Oil Inventory

NAME	USED FOR	DATE OPENED	FAVORITE?

Essential Oil Wish List

NAME	USED FOR	PRICE	KID SAFE?

Printed in Poland
by Amazon Fulfillment
Poland Sp. z o.o., Wrocław

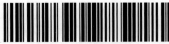